Back to Health

*Lake Worth Chiropractor Reveals Secrets to
Keeping Your Back and Body Healthy*

Craig Selinger, D.C.

Medical Illustrations by Grayson LaPayover

First Printing, 2010
ISBN: 1456449907
ISBN-13: 9781456449902

Printed in the United States of America

For Harriet Selinger,
a mom, inspiration, and the greatest cheerleader
someone could have in their corner. Thanks.

TABLE OF CONTENTS

Purpose i

Introduction. iii

Chapter 1 Spinal anatomy 101 1

Chapter 2 Types of injuries 7

Chapter 3 Changing your lifestyle. 9

Chapter 4 Maintance. 15

Chapter 5 Sports and Exercise 23

Chapter 6 Ergonomics. 41

Chapter 7 Chores 49

Chapter 8 Travel tips 51

Chapter 9 Wrapping it up 61

MEDICAL DISCLAIMER PAGE

Any information given is to be used for educational and information purposes only. It should never be substituted for the medical advice from your own doctor or other health care professionals.

Readers should consult appropriate health professionals on any matter relating to their health and well-being.

The information and opinions provided here are believed to be accurate and sound, based on the best judgment available to the author, but readers who fail to consult appropriate health authorities assume the risk of any injuries. This book is not a substitute for medical treatment or chiropractic care.

THE PURPOSE OF THIS BOOK

I became a chiropractor to help people. The purpose of this book is to motivate and educate people on the importance of spinal health. I have some comic undertones in the book because humor helps people remember concepts and ideas.

I want people to take responsibility for their health and well-being. When people strengthen their body, they are less susceptible to back injuries. Many people take better care of their car than themselves. A healthy spine can improve a person's quality of life. I realize that many people who read this book suffer with low back pain. Before doing the exercises in the book, make sure you consult your health care provider.

ABOUT THE AUTHOR

Craig Selinger, D.C. practices chiropractic in Lake Worth, Florida. He lives in Boca Raton, Florida. Graduated from SUNY Binghamton in 1991 then attended Life Chiropractic College and graduated in 1996. He enjoys stand-up comedy, skiing, surfing, and traveling.

He can be contacted at 561-434-9949 or found on the web at www.mylakeworthchiropractor.com

INTRODUCTION

The thought of writing a book was scary. I thought it would be an impossible task. But then I thought of another person who recently wrote two books: Sarah Palin. Sarah Palin wrote a book that sold 700,000 copies in the first week. She wrote a book because, I guess, she felt she couldn't fit enough information on her hand. I thought, If Sarah Palin can write a book, then I could too. I wrote this book because I felt my experience and training could make a difference in a person's life. Imagine waking up and not being able to get out of bed. In May 2010, this happened to me. I didn't have back pain. I had intense abdominal pain and was dehydrated. After many tests, I was admitted to the hospital. I was later diagnosed with colitis. When I was sick, all I wanted was to be healthy again. When I was well, I took my health for granted. Being ill made me realized the importance of my health. Everything stopped when I was ill: Work, relationships, eating, and exercise.

It's not fun being in the hospital—bad food, loud noise, and weird roommates. Two places you don't get to choose your roommates are hospitals and prison. They put you with people who have different illnesses. So you end up catching something else. You go in with colitis and you come out with pneumonia. My hospital roommate's breathing respirator was so loud I thought Darth Vader was stalking me. In the morning I woke up to a needle in my arm, people running down the hall half naked wearing gowns, and a sixty-year-old roommate high on pain meds, I thought I was in LA, but it wasn't a dream. Lucky for me, my condition could be controlled, and I soon recovered. Thank God I recovered. I'm also thankful for health insurance. It was over $5000 per day to stay at the hospital. I hope these politicians get healthcare reform right. Soon, the only place people are going to be able to afford to have their x-rays taken is at the airport.

After this experience of being sick, I became passionate about educating people about health and wellness.

What would happen if you couldn't work or drive your kids to school? Your health is your most precious resource. Without your health, you can't enjoy your life. Nothing else matters unless you have your health.

It's possible to be healthier and enjoy a better quality of life regardless of your age or circumstance. People have had miraculous recoveries from disease and disability. The best way to avoid disease and disability is to take proactive measures to be healthy. Taking steps to improve your health gives you a fighting chance at a better life.

"You miss 100% of the shots you don't take." –Wayne Gretzky.

I love that quote. Do whatever it takes; step up to be healthy. There are no guarantees in life, except guaranteed failure if we don't try. "Keep shooting!" Do whatever it takes to be healthy. Having a healthy back is part of having a healthy lifestyle.

Quality of life is key. What kind of life to do you have? Can you do the things you want?

Lower back conditions rob people of their independence and quality of life.

Before we discuss ways to achieve a healthy back, we need to understand the anatomy of the back and nervous system. Learning about the anatomy of the spine will help us understand what structures of the spine need to be strengthened.

CHAPTER 1

Spinal Anatomy 101

What structures make up the back?

The back is part of your lower spine. The spine protects the spinal cord. The brain and spinal cord make up the central nervous system. The central nervous system controls and coordinates all the functions of the body directly or indirectly. Messages from the brain travel down the spinal cord through spinal nerves to the rest of the body. Nerve signals also travel back to the brain providing feedback to the brain.

The brain and spinal cord directs the organs, muscles, and glands, the same way a movie director directs a film, but the brain doesn't have to deal with huge egos or with people that need to be in rehab.

The central nervous system is the master controller of the body and the most important system in the body, so it must be protected. The skull encases the brain, and the spinal column protects the spinal cord. The spinal column or "backbone" protects the spinal cord. The spinal column is made up of twenty-four movable small bones called vertebrae.

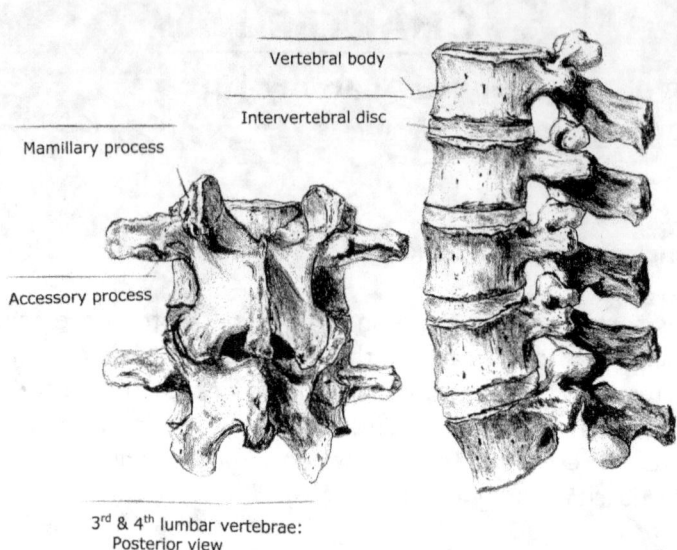

Lumbar vertebrae, assembled:
Left lateral view

Vertebral body

Intervertebral disc

Mamillary process

Accessory process

3rd & 4th lumbar vertebrae:
Posterior view

This is an illustration of a vertebral body and an intervertebral disc. These vertebrae are stacked up on one another and form the spinal column. Between each vertebra is a little "shock absorber" called an intervertebral disc. Ligaments, discs, and muscles hold the vertebra in place. There is a hole in each vertebra, and the spinal cord runs through this hole called the "spinal canal." The spinal cord is surrounded by bone; this is called the spinal canal. Nerves branch off at each vertebral level. After nerves branch off, they go to other parts of the body. The top seven vertebral segments make up the neck or cervical spine. The next twelve vertebras make up the mid back or the thoracic spine. The lower five vertebras make up the low back or lumbar spine. The lumbar spine holds most of the body's weight. (Need a martini yet? We're almost through with the science stuff…hang in there.)

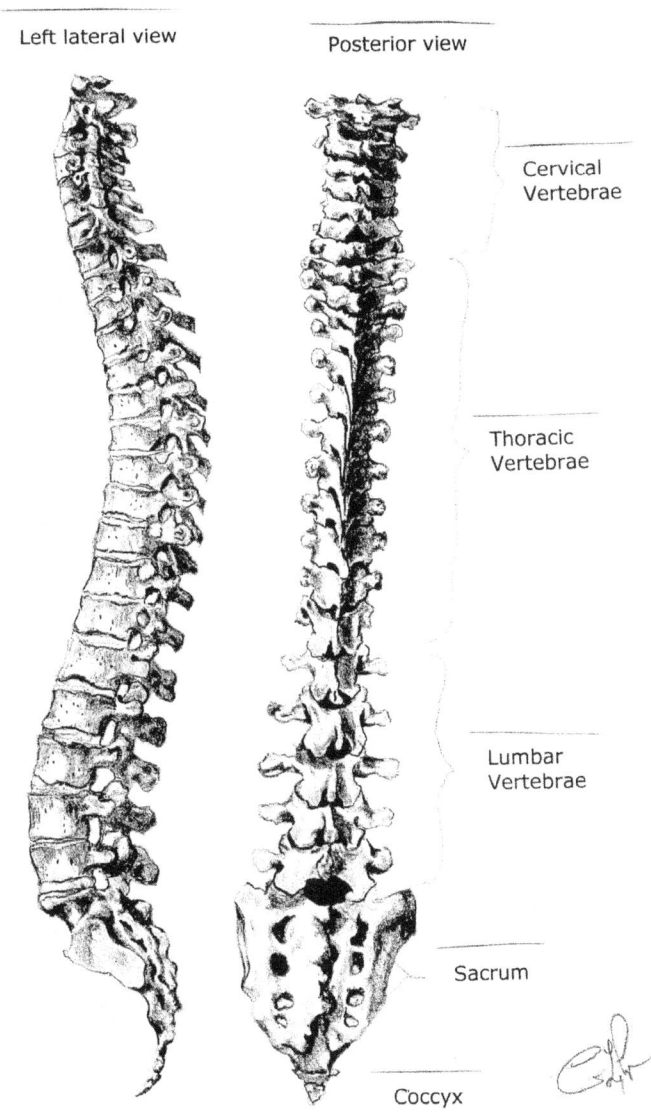

Left lateral view

Posterior view

Cervical
Vertebrae

Thoracic
Vertebrae

Lumbar
Vertebrae

Sacrum

Coccyx

The spine is a strong weight bearing structure. If we look at the spine from the front to back, it should be straight. From the side view, we have three curves: an inward curve in the neck, an outward curve in the mid back, and an inward curve in the low back.

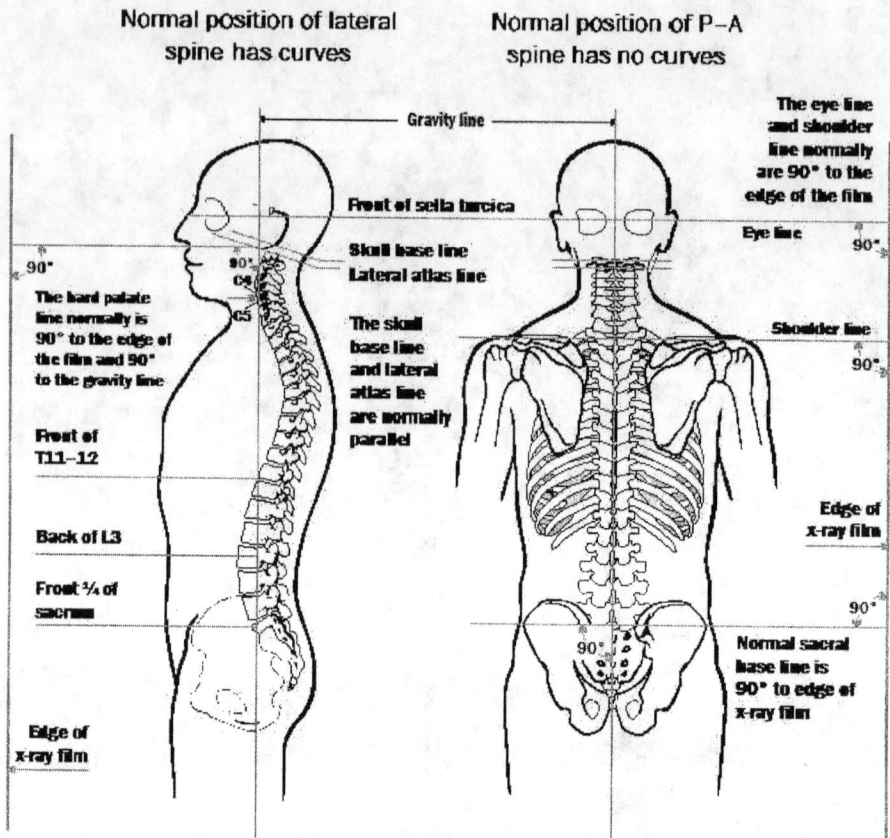

Normal position of lateral spine has curves

Normal position of P–A spine has no curves

Gravity line

The eye line and shoulder line normally are 90° to the edge of the film

Front of sella turcica

Eye line

90°

Skull base line
Lateral atlas line

90°

C9
C5

The hard palate line normally is 90° to the edge of the film and 90° to the gravity line

The skull base line and lateral atlas line are normally parallel

Shoulder line

90°

Front of T11–12

Back of L3

Edge of x-ray film

Front ¾ of sacrum

90°

90°

Normal sacral base line is 90° to edge of x-ray film

Edge of x-ray film

If you look at the illustration of the vertebral column, you will see how the spine should look from a side view, lateral view, and a back view of the spine. The curves in the spine act as shock absorbers, protecting from the impact of walking and other activities. The small discs of the spine are compressed each time a person bends or moves. If the spinal nerves or spinal cord become compressed, the nerve messages will not reach their intended destination. That means messages will not reach the organ, gland, or muscle. This results in a miscommunication between the brain and the rest of the body, which leads to dysfunction and later disease. Just like miscommunications can cause the breakdown of a reality TV star.

A herniated disc, tumor, bone spur, or misaligned vertebra can put pressure on the spinal cord or spinal nerves.

Sometimes when a nerve is compressed, we feel pain, numbness, or muscle weakness; however, not all nerves in the spine sense pain, so you can a have a compressed nerve and not feel it.

What is Low Back Pain?

Low back pain is a symptom. Symptoms are warning signs that something is wrong. A symptom is like the oil warning light in the car. It's a sign of a problem. But the oil light itself is not the true problem; the problem is the car needing oil. After the oil is changed, the light goes off. Once the cause of the low back pain is handled, the symptoms go away.

Low back pain is a common symptom of a low back injury, but it can also be caused by disease, infection, spinal tumors, failed back surgery, pelvic inflammatory disease, aortic aneurysm, peptic ulcers, urinary disorders (kidney stones or urinary tract infections), prostate disease, or a drunken fall. In this book we are going to address low back pain being caused by injury.

Back conditions are endemic in our society. According to *Newsweek* in 2005, Americans spent $85.9 billion on back and neck pain, up from 52.1 billion reported in a 1997 (*Journal of the American Medical Association*). Nearly 65 million Americans report a recent episode of back pain. Back pain is the 6th most costly condition in the United States, according to *Health Affairs* "The most expensive medical conditions in America." Every year, 150 million workdays are lost due to back pain (reported in *To Your Health Magazine*). The Bureau of Labor Statistics reports that 1 in every 5 injuries in the workplace account for back injuries. There are also secondary effects of back conditions. The inability to work and function results in depression. Low back pain can have consequences for the family, leading to job loss and bankruptcy. Back pain sufferers can easily become addicted to pain medication. Even though these medications are sometimes necessary, they can be dangerous and lead to weird behavior.

I had a patient with severe low back pain come into my office; the next day he returned and told me he took pain killers because his pain levels were high. He said he didn't notice anything different. I looked at him and wondered, *Well, did you notice that you that you shaved your eyebrows off?* People on pain medication can do some bizarre things. This is a humorous story, but many stories about people taking pain medication are not funny.

Back injuries are a serious problem, but there are steps we can take to overcome this condition and still keep your eyebrows.

CHAPTER 2
Types of Injuries

Most low back injuries are caused by the following: 1) Material handling: carrying, pulling, lifting, or pushing objects. 2) Trauma: high-speed impact, falling, or being struck by an object. Trauma can cause muscles, ligaments, or a disc to tear. Vertebra may even become fractured. 3) Repetitive injury: an activity that is done over and over can reproduce small injury to muscles, ligaments, or a disc. The activity is typically a repetitive incorrect lifting technique, also known as cumulative trauma disorder. This repetitive activity causes minor damage to structures of the back each time the person performs the activity. Over time, the person has accumulated minor injuries that can become a major injury.

Strained muscles of the low back are the most common injury. Muscles can become strained when they are overworked while doing chores, labor, or during exercise.

A herniated disc is an injury that occurs when the disc tears and the soft disc material inside the disc leaks out. This causes inflammation and often leads to nerves or the spinal cord becoming compressed. "Stenosis" is the spinal nerves or spinal cord becoming compressed. Stenosis means narrowing or constriction. Stenosis can be caused by degeneration of the spine. "Bone spurs" are a build up of calcium deposits can compress nerves or the spinal cord. This condition is common in people who are over sixty years old. Stenosis can also be caused by a tumor, which can put pressure on the spinal cord or spinal nerves as well.

Compensations

Now this is not when an insecure guy goes out and buys a Porsche to build his self-esteem up. The compensations we are talking about are when muscles are overused and become injured. The body will get the help of other muscles to help the injured muscles perform their job. This is called compensation. Eventually, the stronger muscles that have been helping the weaker muscle becomes overworked and then they become weak themselves. This results in an injury to the stronger muscles. This is a common way the low back becomes injured. It's like the weaker muscles are slackers at work, then the other workers on the team have pick up the slack for the slackers. Eventually, the team gets overworked and becomes dysfunctional; they start drinking, showing up late, and start watching *Real Housewives of New Jersey*.

There are things we can do to overcome these injuries. If you strengthen the weak muscles, you can avoid these types of injuries and build a stronger back.

"Doctor every morning when I get up and look in the mirror I feel like throwing up. What's wrong with me? He said, I don't know, but your eyesight is perfect."

— Rodney Dangerfield.

Rodney Dangerfield was one of my favorite comedians. It's important to see a doctor and have your condition properly diagnosed.

Sometimes your condition is obvious, sometimes it's not. Something what seems like a minor problem can be more serious.

It might be an emergency...Call 911 or go the Emergency Room

Back pain can be a sign of a medical emergency. If you or someone experiences the following symptoms, seek immediate medical attention:

- Leg weakness
- Loss of bowel or bladder control
- Unexplained weight loss, loss of appetite with back pain
- Sudden, severe abdominal pain accompanied by low back pain
- Fever with increased low back pain, especially after surgery
- Pain in neck or back with weakness and or numbness in arms or legs
- Back pain that does not improve with rest and gets worse at night

CHAPTER 3

Changing Your Lifestyle

Who runs your life? Twitter?

Facebook runs most people's life. NO, YOU RUN YOUR LIFE! (That's a literary Sam Kinison scream). No doctor or anyone else can take responsibility for your health without you first taking responsibility. Having a strong back and doing certain tasks differently can help you to have a healthy back and a better quality of life. If we took care of our teeth like most of us take care of our backs there would be a lot of toothless people walking around. Well, this is true in some parts in the U.S.

Many people don't know how to take care of their back. This book will give you tips to help you take care of your back. Some people know what they should do, but they don't do it. Many people don't apply what they learn. We need to create new habits to bring about real change. You need to run your life and set your course to be healthy. If you want to have a healthy back, you need to change your lifestyle. Ultimately, you need to be fit and have a healthy lifestyle. Many people in the U.S. are not fit and don't have a healthy lifestyle. If you want to be healthy, you need to take charge and make it happen. Most of the tips I am going to recommend are going to involve making changes to your lifestyle. This can be difficult, so I am going to help you make a plan.

Set Goals…

Things don't happen by accident. Your actions and decisions bring about outcomes. If you want to be in a better place, you need to make better decisions and take the appropriate action. You didn't just wake up one morning fifty pounds overweight. It took a poor diet and lack of exercise. Still, you are responsible. Not doing the right things is a choice.

Outcomes occur in our lives; things happen whether we plan them or not. Outcomes are the results of decisions we make. The decisions were based on a goal. If we make decisions that support reaching our goals, we usually get what we want. When we want something bad enough, we will usually take the steps to get it. However, we take our health for granted. We don't think about our health until we become sick or disabled. Be proactive. Set goals that support our health and form routines or habits to achieve a health life.

For many, the toughest changes will be starting an exercise program and changing your diet. It starts with a goal. Have the end in mind. What kind of body do we want? What do we want to be able to do? Whose wedding do we want to dance at? What color Speedo will we buy? This is an important aspect of being healthy and having a healthy back.

Being fit should be your goal. Many people want to lose weight. I advise people to have SMART (Specific, Measurable, Attainable, Realistic, and Timely) goals. (George T. Doran, 1981)

Being specific makes it easy to understand what desired outcome we want, why we want that outcome, and how we are going to get it.

The next part of goal setting is for the desired result to be measurable. How do we know when we reach the goal? We need to have criteria to measure our progress toward reaching our goal.

Next, the goal must be attainable. Is this a goal that is possible to reach?

Is the goal realistic, is it do-able? Setting the bar too high can discourage people from trying to reach the goal. For example, I could never be able to be a center for the Knicks.

The last important criteria a goal should have is a timeframe. Deadlines are important! We need to know the due date. A good example of a goal would be, "I must lose eighteen pounds by June 25, 2012."

Have a Strong Why...

Why do you want to reach your goal? People need a reason to do things. The more difficult the task, the stronger reasons a person needs to be to reach his/her goal. Visual images can be powerful; images of how you want to look are great for people that want to get fit. Photos of grandkids might motivate you to be healthy for them. Images can motivate you and keep you on course with your program. Visualize how you will look. What will you be able to do? How much better will you feel? Who will you become during the process?

Pain / Pleasure...

Anthony Robbins talks about how pain and pleasure are the chief motivating factors that influence our decision-making. If we associate pain with doing something, we won't do it. People associate more pain to cleaning their closet, so they put it off until they absolutely can't avoid doing it, or their closet starts to smell like sweaty feet. If we associate pleasure to doing something, we'll do it. Pain can be a bigger motivator if we associate pain to not doing something. Use pain to get leverage to motivate you to take action. How will you live if you do become disabled? What will you miss out on?

Make Health a Habit...

"It's not the things we do once in a while that make a difference, it's the things we do everyday."

–Anthony Robbins

Wouldn't it be great to get what we want without having to think about it? Image...automatically completing important tasks that help us reach our goals without thinking about it.

When we do something repeatedly, it can become ingrained in our daily routine. When a task becomes part of our daily routine, it becomes a habit. Wikipedia defines a habit as an acquired pattern of behavior that often occurs automatically. Wouldn't it be great to become healthy automatically? Once these behaviors become part of our everyday lives, they become a quick and easy way to achieve our goals.

Break it down...

No, I'm not talking about MC Hammer. Break goals into achievable short-term goals. If I have a goal to lose five pounds in five months, then I need to break the goal down into parts: lose one pound per month. Then, I need to find out how to lose a pound. I can diet and/or exercise. The action steps to achieving goals are important. If we do the same action steps consistently, our nervous system can get used to this activity. Once we program ourselves to do this activity on a regular basis, it becomes part of our daily routine, like showering and brushing our teeth. I wish everyone had these habits. We just feel like doing it, and we don't have to think about it. This becomes a habit; it becomes automatic.

Start with scheduling this task in your calendar. Walking around the block can become a daily routine that gets to become a habit we just feel like doing, and, if we don't do it, we feel guilty. Use guilt as leverage to achieve your result.

The first tips are going to deal with forming new habits that will help you to have a healthy back.

Here are some ways to transform activities into habits.

1) Look at the reasons why you want the goal. Look at the photos of how you want to look. Develop a strong emotional reason why you must continue with this activity. Each day you do the activity, give yourself a small reward right after you do it. Not a Twinkie, but maybe sushi. Have a calendar and schedule the time you are going to do your new habit. Keep reviewing your goal and

2) Get an activity buddy. No, not to go on play dates, but someone to do the activity with.

3) Have some accountability. You have to set up consequences for not following through. You might set up a fine system. For instance, if you don't do your walk then you will have to pay a small fine to your friend. You and your buddy can play a game. Or you can do the reverse fine system: at the start of the workout program give each other $100. Each day that you are scheduled to work out and you do, your buddy will give you $10; if you work out five days a week in two weeks, you will have the $100 back. However, if you miss a day, your buddy gets to keep the $10 for that day. I like the reverse fine system because you get rewarded for following through. This is a good game because many people will do almost anything to avoid losing money.

Replace it...

If you are cutting something out of your diet or stop doing something like smoking, you need to replace that activity with something else. Now that you are not consuming as many sweets and soda, you can replace it with fruits, vegetables, and water. Unfortunately, when many people stop smoking they replace smoking with eating or drinking. This is difficult. My goal is not to turn you into an obese, uptight alcoholic. Replace the bad habit with something that is healthy.

Don't be too hard on yourself…keep at…

Lifestyle changes can be difficult. Try small changes first, then take on more change. If you mess up, don't give up! Get back and try again.

Be in a good environment…

If you surround yourself with healthy people, you will probably become healthier. If you go to the gym on a regular basis and socialize with people who are working out, you will become like them. And the reverse is also true. If you want to stop drinking then don't hang out in Hollywood, chances are you'll need to be in an intervention program.

CHAPTER 4

Maintenance

The body is like a car, if you want it to run well you need to maintain it. Having a strong body is a good way to fight off disease and disability. A weaker body is more susceptible to injury and disease.

Tip 1 – See a Chiropractor

The Chinese have been doing spinal manipulation for thousands of years. "Tui Na" is the Chinese art of manipulation of the spine and other joints to restore health. Spinal manipulation was rediscovered and refined in the United States. Chiropractic has refined the art, philosophy, and science of spinal manipulation.

Chiropractic began in the United States and was founded by Daniel David Palmer in 1895 in Davenport, Iowa. Daniel David Palmer was a healer. In September 1895, he treated a janitor named Harvey Lillard, who had been deaf for seventeen years. He saw a large lump in Mr. Lillard's spine. This man's spine was grossly out of alignment. He applied firm pressure to the spine with his hands. After that, miraculously the man could hear. He thought he discovered a cure for deafness, so hundreds of people who were deaf were treated. Unfortunately, no other patients regained their hearing; however, patients saw other changes: one man had success with heart trouble while other people had experienced improvement with other health conditions.

"Chiropractic" comes from the Greek word Chiropraktikos, meaning "effective treatment by hand."

Later, B.J. Palmer, the son of Daniel David Palmer, developed chiropractic into a healing art, science, and philosophy. Chiropractic was based on the following principles:

- Chiropractic was based on the body's ability to heal itself without the use of drugs or surgery.
- Good health relies on having a normally functioning nervous system.
- The body will not function properly when there is interference of nerve impulses between the brain and the body.

Chiropractic helped many people with neck and back conditions, but it is not limited to neck and back pain. A recent study conducted by George Bakris, M.D., director of the hypertension center at the University of Chicago Medical Center, conducted a placebo-controlled study that demonstrated a decrease in blood pressure from those patients that received chiropractic treatment. What other things can chiropractic help with?

Chiropractic can also help your spine last longer. If the front end of your car were out of alignment, how would the tires wear? They would wear out faster and would wear out unevenly. Then your tire would blow out and you would crash. (Sorry for the unpleasant analogy, they get better later on.)

When the spine is misaligned, it causes increased wear and tear on the spine; a misaligned spine degenerates faster than a non-misaligned spine. Chiropractors help correct these misalignments and help restore proper nerve flow. With proper nerve flow, the body can function better.

Tip 2 – Acupuncture

For thousands of years the Chinese have been using acupuncture to treat over 2000 health conditions. Acupuncture is a system of healing that involves stimulating points on the skin to treat the body. Acupuncture is based on helping to balance the energy of the body known as "Chi" or "Qi". This energy flows through the body along pathways called meridians. If the flow of Qi is blocked, dysfunction, pain, or illness can occur. By stimulating acupuncture points around the body, normal energy flows can be restored. Acupuncture, like chiropractic, should be part of a person's wellness routine. Acupuncture should be done to keep your body healthy. Acupuncture can help a person to have balanced Qi, which can help keep us well. I wish they had an acupuncture point to cure Facebook addiction.

Tip 3 – Bodywork or Massage

Bodywork and massage can help to unwind tight muscles, help with posture, relax the body, and rehabilitate injured muscles. When muscles are injured, scare tissue forms in the muscle. Scar tissue can limit the function of the muscle. Some types of body work and massage can help breakdown the scar tissue and help the body form new muscle tissue in the affected area.

Rolfing

Over fifty years ago, Dr. Rolf developed a system of bodywork with its aim to release tight muscles and realign and balance the posture. Rolfers work on stretching the fascia. Fascia is tissue that surrounds and connects muscles, blood vessels, and nerves. When the fascia is too restrictive it can alter muscle function. Rolfers try to stretch this fascia to help ease tension though out the body to enhance function.

Egoscue

Is a system of stretches and exercises custom tailored to each person's posture and muscle tone.

Massage Therapy

Massage relieves tension, can help increase flexibility, and increase circulation and blood flow to an area. When there is more blood flow to an area, faster healing will occur. Massage can help release endorphins, which are the body's natural pain relievers. Massage therapy breaks down scar tissue and releases muscles from spasms. It is becoming more recognized as a form of medical treatment; a study by the American Massage Therapy Association found that 54% of healthcare providers encourage massage therapy.

Tip 4 – Get Out of Bed Properly

Did you know you could hurt your back just by getting out of bed each day? Getting out of bed improperly can cause strain on your back. When you get out of bed, roll on your side, and then bend both legs at the knees, put legs over the side of the bed. Push using your hands against the bed and swing your legs down. Now in the sitting position, push up off the bed. Go to www.mylakeworthchiropractor.com for a video demonstration.

Tip 5 - Lose Weight

"This morning when I put on my underwear I could hear the fruit-of-the-loom guys laughing at me."

–Rodney Dangerfield

People are not honest with themselves about losing weight; they don't think it's a problem. "Yeah, Bob, your belly is supposed to extend out and go six inches below your belt buckle. That's great, now your feet don't get wet when it rains."

The excess weight puts more stress on the spine. Many overweight people develop osteoarthritis because of the increased wear and tear on their spine.

The excess weight contributes to poor posture, which causes muscles to work overtime just to maintain a relaxed posture. The result is chronic muscle fatigue and muscle tightness.

Being overweight and sedentary causes low back conditions. The muscles remain weak from inactivity. When the person does minimal activity, they experience pain and later can develop osteoporosis, a weakening of the bones.

I advise patients to adopt the zone diet developed by Dr. Barry Sears, which is based on eating carbohydrates, proteins, and fats in the proper ratio, 40:30:30. That means 40% carbohydrates, 30% protein, and 30% fats. This ratio has been shown to be a effective dietary approach. Stay away from eating refined carbo-hydrates, like white pasta, white rice, and white breads. A diet high in refined carbohydrates causes a sharp rise and fall in glucose levels. The sharp rise in glucose levels causes a sharp rise in insulin levels. This may lead to diabetes and other health related conditions. A diet high in refined carbohydrate is a recipe for packing on major weight.

Losing weight is basic math. If you use or burn up more calories than you consume, you will lose weight. To maintain your weight, the average man has to consume about 2500 calories per day, the average woman about 2000 calories per day (2500 calories in third trimester of pregnancy), and 1800 calories for children five to ten years old. These are average calorie amounts to maintain your weight. To lose weight, you will need to consume less than this amount or burn more calories by exercising. To get a more accurate calorie count that is right for you, go to free dieting the weight loss guide's website below. Plug in your age, gender, height, weight, and amount of times you exercise. This site will help you calculate your own calorie budget. If you consume more than this amount you will gain weight and if you consume less than this amount you will lose weight.

http://www.freedieting.com/tools/calorie_calculator.htm

There are many new helpful tools to lose weight. "Lose it," is the name of an iPhone application that can tell you the calorie content of foods you consume. Knowing the amount of calories you consume daily can give you an idea of how much you consume versus how much you should consume. You can have a budget for calories you consume. You burn more calories when you exercise. Consuming fewer calories in your diet and exercising means you take in less and burn more. This is the fastest way to lose weight. Also, when you build muscle, your metabolism increases; a faster metabolism means you burn more calories when you are RESTING. Cool, huh?

Lose It has a large database of brand name foods, even the ones you shouldn't eat like Chef Boyardee and McDonalds. Search the database for the foods you eat, your portion size, and add it to your breakfast, lunch, dinner, or snack log.

Exercise is also factored into your Lose It daily caloric allowance. The amount of calories burned is added onto your daily calorie maximum. Go to http://www.loseit.com "step trak lite" is another iPhone application that can help you be fit. This application will count the number of steps you take and how long you run or walk for.

"Ishape" is another iPhone application that lets you track calories and monitor exercise.

Tip 6 - Stress Management

Stress can cause many health problems, one being muscle spasms. Muscle spasms can occur when we overreact to a situation and our muscles become over stimulated remaining in the contracted position. Stress management techniques like mediation, exercise, tai chi, vacations, chiropractic, massage, acupuncture, or counseling can help us deal with the stress. We will be less likely to have low back pain after our muscles relax.

Tip 7 - Meditation

In an overstressed environment, having tools to calm the mind and body can help us stay sane. Meditation is a technique to calm the mind and the body. There are many different forms of meditation. Just ten to fifteen minutes of breathing exercises keeping our back straight and focusing our mind on breathing. That's right—try to stay focused on breathing in and out. Preferably, breathe through the nose. You can sit in a chair or sit cross-legged. Just keep the back straight.

Go to this site to learn how to mediate. Just don't meditate while driving, instead of becoming one with the universe you'll become one with a Prius.

Go to Youtube and check the video John Kabat-Zinn made while doing a presentation at Google:

http://www.youtube.com/watch?v=3nwwKbM_vJc

Tip 8 - Stop Smoking

Research shows that smokers are more likely than non-smokers to develop back pain. Not only does smoking make you look older, it can lead to back pain. And watch out Marlboro man smoking causes impotency too.

Smoking can clog up the arteries that supply blood and oxygen to the lower spine. This deteriorates the spinal disks. Smoking can interfere with the body's ability to deliver nutrients to the discs of the spine. With insufficient nutrients, the tissues of the back can't repair when damaged, which later results in back aches.

- Nicotine from cigarettes can affect the way the brain senses pain.
- Smoking can cause heavy coughing that can cause back pain.
- Smoking slows down the healing process; this slows down the repair of low back.
- Smoking also causes impotency.

Treatment

Stop smoking…whether you use medicine, acupuncture, or hypnosis. Just do it. When you stop smoking, your body will start to repair, even if you have been smoking for years.

Tip 9 - The Hot Tub

James Brown sang about the hot tub, because they're awesome to relieve sore, tight muscles. Hot tubs can be a great way to loosen tight muscles. The hot water helps increase circulation and blood flow to tight, contracted muscles. I would not stay in longer than fifteen minutes at a time. The temperature should not exceed 104 degrees Fahrenheit. People with high blood pressure, heart disease, diabetes, pregnant women, and those people that pass out easily should see their doctor before going into a hot tub.

Tip 10 - Try Infrared Heat

Infrared heat can help to heal. It's like actual light waves that heat, like the sun.

Tip 11 - Be Careful of Medication Side Effects

Some medications cause side effects that might include low back or neck pain. A common side of effect of Statins is muscle pain and or muscle weakness.

Prednisone is a medication used to treat many inflammatory conditions, especially IBS, colitis, and crohn's disease. This medication can cause muscle cramps and/or pain. Make sure you know the side effects of the medications you are taking.

CHAPTER 5

Exercise and Sports

Tip 12 – Exercise: "it's not a four letter word"

When you say the word "exercise" in some places people look at you like you said a four-letter word. The word "exercise," is so shocking to most people it's as shocking as Keith Richards walking in a straight line, god bless him. Exercise not only helps us live longer and healthier, it can also help with many back conditions. Weak back muscles are a major cause of low back pain. Stronger back muscles will be able to sustain more stress and not become easily injured.

I recommend exercising five days per week for at least thirty minutes. Do a variety of exercises and incorporate exercises that strengthen the abdominals and the low back. Exercises that involve bending the torso forward and backward help to strengthen the low back and the abdominals. I recommend that beginners take an exercise class at their gym prior to starting an exercise program. Exercises that are done incorrectly can lead to injury.

Stretching is also important. Many injuries occur because muscles are not flexible and tear when they are overexerted. Stretching allows muscles to be able to move through a full range of motion; it releases tension and helps the body move properly. If one muscle is too tight, another muscle will have to lend a hand to help that tighten muscle do its job.

Stretching the hamstrings, gluts, and quadriceps (muscles in the buttocks, back of the leg, and front of the leg) can help to alleviate stress on the low back. Tight hamstrings can act as an anchor weighting the low back down. This pulling effect can lead to low back pain and sciatica (pain down the leg).

Check out these sites for stretching demonstration:

http://www.youtube.com/watch?v=BaDXNjFjjnU

http://www.youtube.com/watch?v=LmBp05_DMrQ

http://www.youtube.com/watch?v=-iY5V0xiiKw

Tip 13 – Weight Training

Weight training involves lifting weights. Lifting weights helps build muscle. Building muscle is great for your spine, but it has many other health benefits. When we build muscle, it also increases our metabolism. We burn fat faster and our body functions better. There are many different weight-training programs. I like full body workouts. That type of workout works large muscle groups and many muscles at one time. I recommend changing your workout routine from time to time. You will work a variety of muscles and keep from getting bored. You can get a great work out in under an hour. Before working out, warm up and do some cardio (treadmill, bicycle, or stair climber) for about five to ten minutes. Then stretch the large muscle groups you will be working. Your first set of your work out should be a light set. To find a variety of workout routines go to:

- Menshealth.com
- Mensfitness.com
- Womenshealthmag.com

The first two weeks of starting an exercise program is the most likely time for injuries. Take it easy and lift less than you think you can lift. When you begin your exercise program, get a personal trainer to properly instruct you how to do the exercises correctly. A weight room injury will suspend your workout routine. So please use light weights and get proper instruction.

Tip: Danger signs associated with exercise are listed below.

If you experience any of these signs, you should seek medical attention:

- Unusual fatigue
- Nausea
- Dizziness
- Tightness or pain in the chest
- Lightheadedness

- Loss of muscle control
- Severe breathlessness
- Allergic reactions (e.g., rash or hives)
- Blurring of vision
- Or thinking that Jersey Shore is a good T.V. show

Dr. Selinger's 10 favorite exercises (don't overdo them!). This is not a program about hurting people so they come to my office. Pick four different exercises each day. Every third day, go back to the exercise you did on the first day. These exercises are designed for relatively fit people. If you have any doubts about being able to do these exercises, see your physician first.

1. **Squats**

Squats help to strengthen many muscles at once. They help to strengthen your glutes (the buttocks), quads, hamstrings, and calves. They also help with your balance. If you have knee injuries skip this exercise. Remember, use lighter weights (ten pounds) or no weight.

To do a squat : Stand a little wider than shoulders width apart, toes facing straight ahead. Slowly bend the knees and lower hips towards the floor, keeping your torso straight and abs pulled in tight. Keep your knees behind your toes; make sure everything's pointing in the same direction. Do not go lower than ninety degrees. Do this exercise every three days for ten to twelve reps. Three sets. You do not need to use weights. Try this exercise without weights. If you want more of a challenge, hold the squat in the down position for one to two seconds then rise up. Light weights can be used, but doing squats with heavy weight can cause damage to the lower back. If you are having difficulty, don't use weights, just practice the form and use a countertop or railing to hold on to so you can do the motion. Another exercise you can do if the squat is too difficult is chair squats. Slowly sit down in a chair and then slowly stand up without using the armrests; this can help build muscles that you use while squatting, and they are easier to do than squats. If you still have difficulty, use the armrest to keep up out the chair. WARNING: MAKE SURE THE ARMREST CAN SUPPORT YOU, AND THE CHAIR IS STURDY. WE DON'T WANT YOU TO FALL.

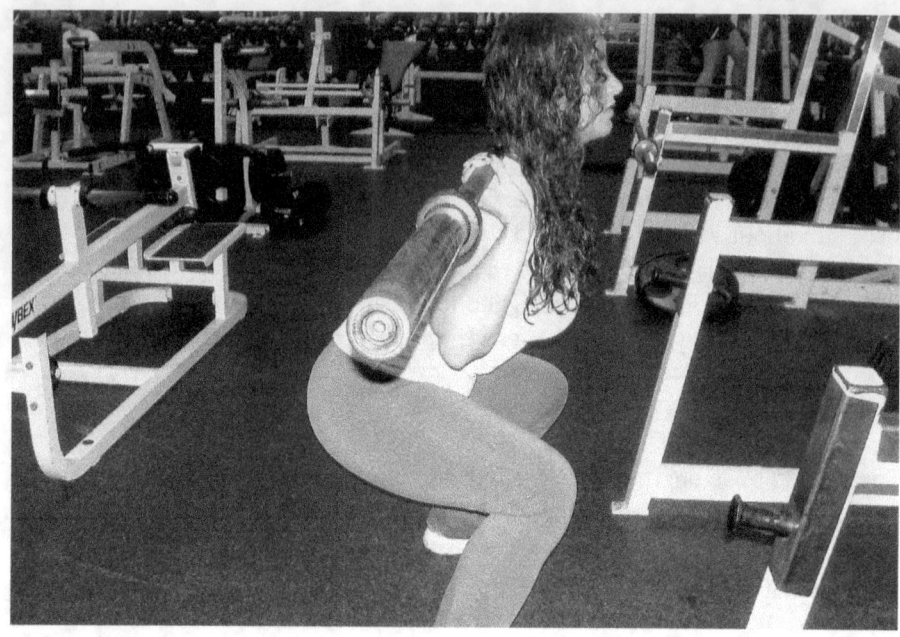

Check out this YouTube video:

http://www.youtube.com/watch?v=acRdlwx1Hh8&feature=fvst

2. **Push-Ups**

Push-ups strengthen many muscles at once. The chest, shoulders, triceps, back, and abs. are strengthened. I would recommend doing these push ups while balancing on your knees first, not on your toes.

To do a push-up: Position yourself face down on the floor, balancing on your toes/knees and hands. Your hands should be wider than shoulders and body in a straight line from head to toe. Don't sag in the middle and don't stick your butt up in the air. Slowly bend your arms and lower your body to the floor, stopping when your elbows are at ninety degrees. Exhale and push back up. Variations include incline, decline or wall pushups. Do this exercise every three days. Do three sets of ten reps. Each week, try to add one rep until you get to fifty push-ups.

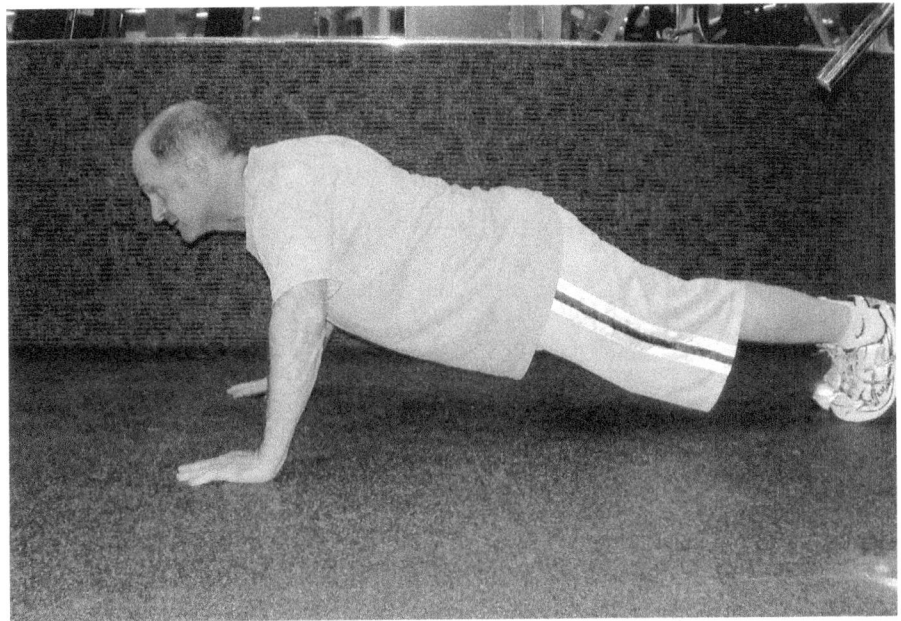

Check out this you tube video:

http://www.youtube.com/watch?v=BbDcMfu-i4w&feature=related

If you suffer from low back pain, try incline push ups. Incline push-ups are easier on your back. Keep your feet on the floor and put your hands on a bench or chair. This takes some pressure off the low back. You still work the chest and triceps. Do the push-ups slowly. If you still experience pain, you can do push-ups while leaning forward on a wall.

Check out this YouTube video:

http://www.youtube.com/watch?v=Z0bRiVhnO8Q

3. Lunges

Lunges strengthens your quads, hamstrings, glutes, and calves.

To do a lunge, stand in a split-stance (one leg forward, one leg back). Bend knees and lower body into a lunge position, keeping the front knee and back knee at ninety-degree angle. Keeping the weight in your heels, and push back up (slowly!) to starting position. Be careful not to lock your knees at the top, and don't let your knee bend past your toes. Do this exercise every three days.

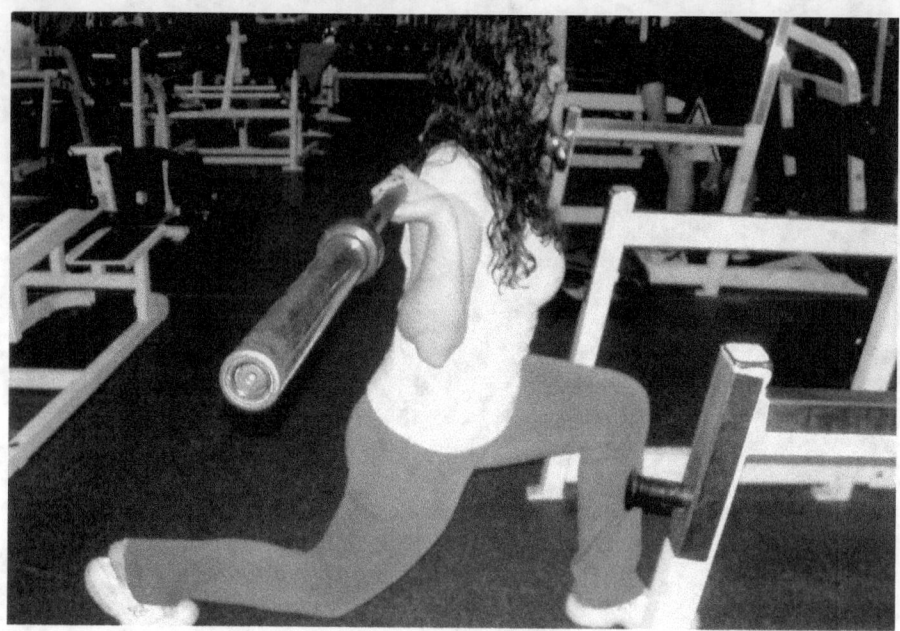

Check out this video on YouTube:

http://www.youtube.com/watch?v=HacUpgo8h80

4. The Plank (Don't worry you don't have to dress like a Pirate)

The plank strengthens the abs, back, arms, and legs all at once.

To do the plank, lie face down on mat with elbows resting on the floor next to your chest. Push your body off the floor in a push-up position with body resting on elbows or hands. Contract the abs and keep the body in a straight line from head to toes. Hold for thirty to sixty seconds and repeat as many times as you can, up to two sets of ten reps. For beginners, do this move on your knees and gradually work your way up to balancing on your toes.

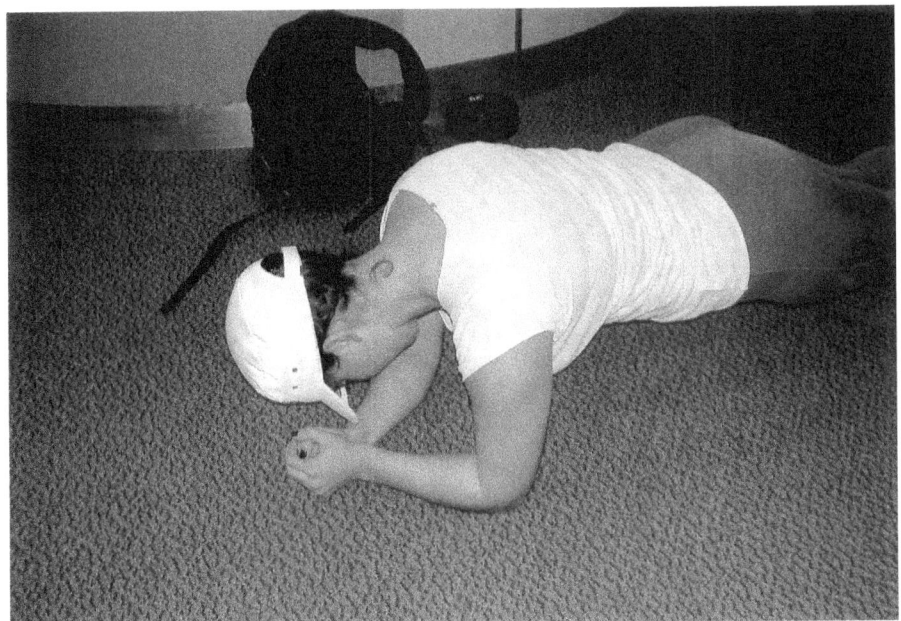

Check out the YouTube video:

http://www.youtube.com/watch?v=MHQmRINu4jU

5. Lat Pull down / or Pull ups

The lat pull down strengthens the major muscles of your back, the latissmus dorsi.

To do a lat pull down, sit on the lat pull down machine and hold the bar with palms out and wider than shoulders. Pull your abs in and lean back slightly. Bend your elbows and pull the bar down towards your chin, contracting the outer muscles of your back. Bring the bar in front of your chin. I recommend not bringing the bar behind your head; this can cause a rotator cuff injury. Do this exercise for three sets of ten.

If you are strong enough, you can do pull-ups. To do pull-ups, hold the pull-up bar palms down a little wider than shoulders width apart and lift your body up till your nose is even with the bar.

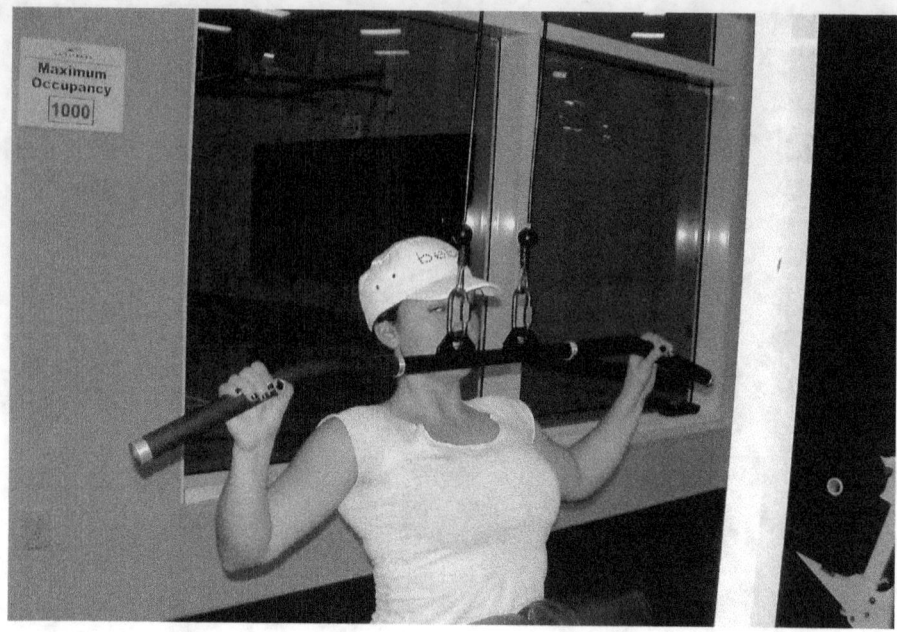

Check out this YouTube video:

http://www.youtube.com/watch?v=EA78cNfUcFA

6. Do Crunches and 86 the Sit-ups

Sit-ups involve using more muscle groups than crunches, but doing sit-ups increases the risk of injuring your low back. Doing crunches strengthens your abdominal muscles and it's a less risky activity than doing full sit-ups.

To do a crunch, lie flat on your back with your knees bent and your feet together flat on the floor and about ten to fifteen inches from your buttocks. Your hands should either be crossed on your chest, by your side, or cupped behind your ears. Without moving your lower body, curl your upper torso up and in toward your knees, until your shoulder blades are as high off the ground as you can. Only your shoulder blades should lift off the ground, not your back. As you come to the highest point, tighten and flex your abdominals for a brief second. Slowly lower yourself back to the starting position. Repeat for reps.

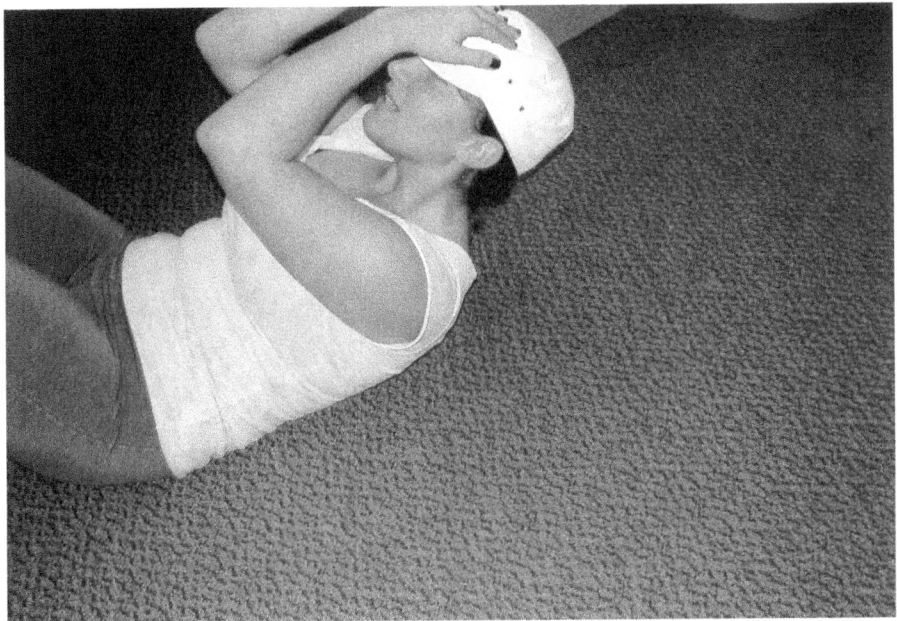

Check out this YouTube video:

http://www.youtube.com/watch?v=i0qh-2haLJQ

7. Shoulder Press with Dumbbells

The shoulder press exercise is excellent for the shoulders and triceps. I recommend using dumbbells. Use light weights.

To do a shoulder press, sit or stand, keeping your back straight. Your shoulders should be back. If you stand, stand a little wider than shoulders width apart; your arms should be bent holding the weights above the chest. Then push your arms up toward the ceiling, bringing them together over your head. If you are advanced, you can combine the shoulder press with the squat to get a more whole body exercise.

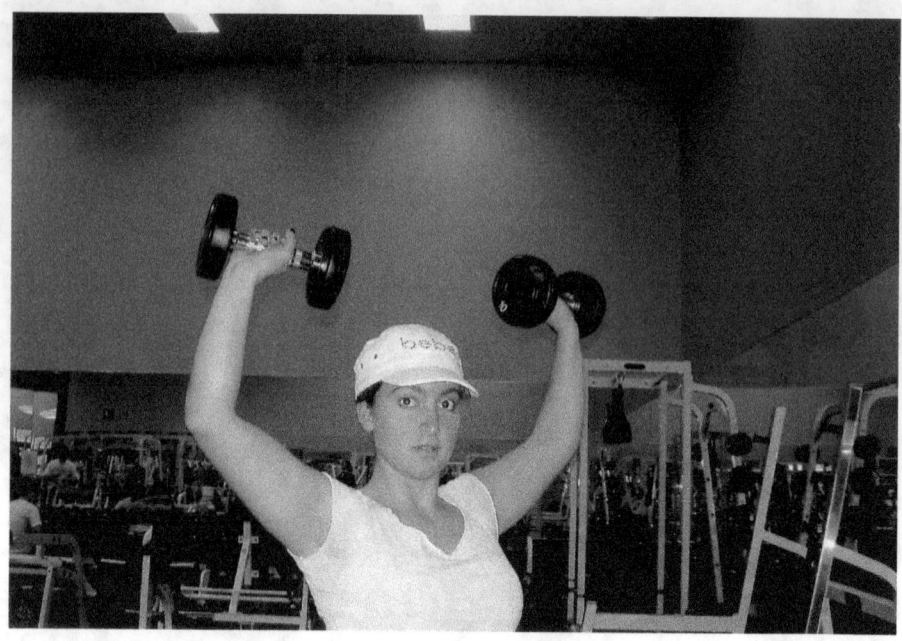

Check out this YouTube video.

http://www.youtube.com/watch?v=YrVsE3hblUc

8. The Superman

This exercise is great for strengthening your mid back, low back, and buttocks. Lie face down on the floor.

To do this exercise, put your hands out in front of you. Lift up your hands and head. Hold your arms and head up for a half a second. Then while your hands are down, raise your legs up. For more of a challenge, raise your hands, head, and legs up at the same time, hold for a half a second.

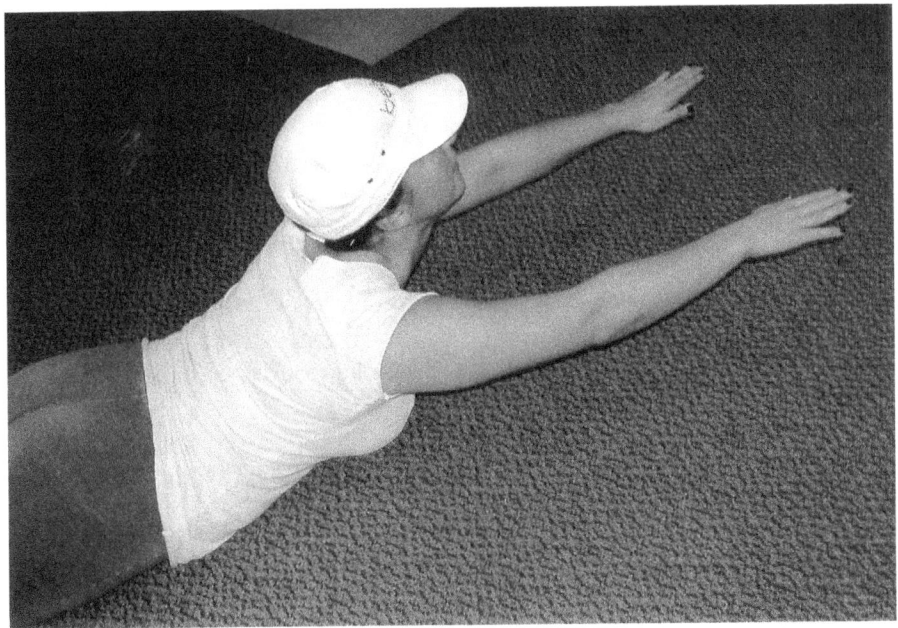

Check out this video on YouTube:

http://www.youtube.com/watch?v=cc6UVRS7PW4&feature=channel

(Do on a day you are not doing the plank.)

9. **Leg Raises**

Great to strengthen the lower abdominal muscles.

To do this exercise, lay on your back with your knees slightly bent, lift your legs about sixty degrees off the floor, then lower your legs to the floor. If this is too difficult, bend your knees more, this exercise is easier if you don't lift your feet off the floor too much. On the next YouTube video, there are some other exercises you can do to strengthen the lower abs. There are different variations of leg raises. Lying on your back while on a mat is the easiest.

1. Lie on your back on an exercise mat. If you put your hands under your where the low back meets the buttock, it's easier.
2. Slightly raise your shoulders and feet off the floor (keep a slight bend in your knees). This is the starting position.

3. Using your abs, raise your legs to approx. Thirty to sixty degrees off the floor. Keep the rest of your body steady.
4. Then slowly lower your legs back to the starting position (try not letting them touch the floor).
5. Repeat until you complete your reps.

Tips:

- Exhale as you lift, inhale as you lower.
- Keep your lower back touching the floor and your neck neutral (don't let your chin move up or down) throughout.
- Focus on bracing your core and keeping your body balanced with a neutral back.

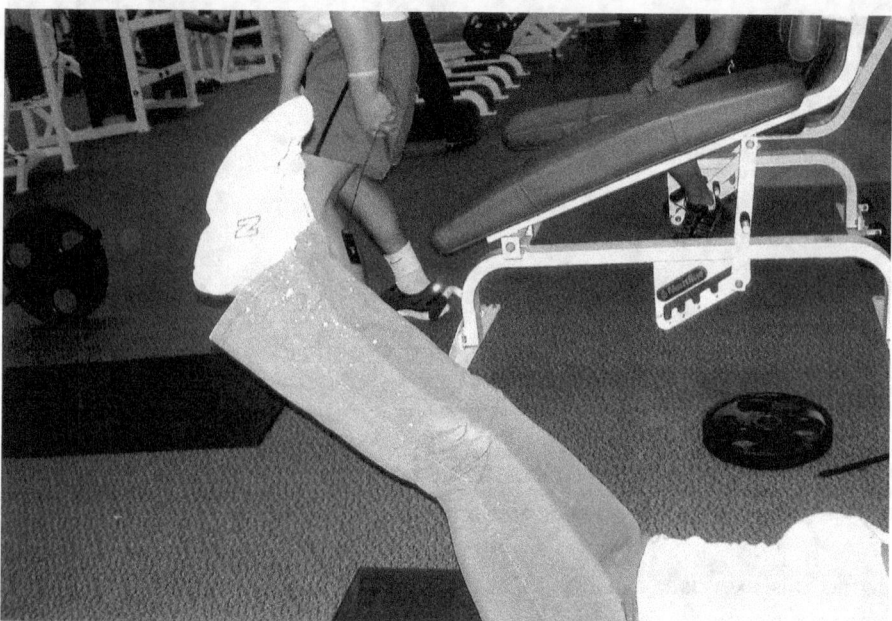

Watch this YouTube video:

http://www.youtube.com/watch?v=MDJ-iLyeOow

10. **Deadlifts.** (No this does not have anything to do with the movie Twilight)

Deadlifts strengthen your back, legs, and forearms. Pull the barbell from the floor with both hands until your body is fully extended. Deadlift, by pushing from the heels, and bringing your hips forward. Not by pulling with your lower back. Don't move the bar to get into proper position. Walk to the bar and position your feet correctly. Then, grab the bar and deadlift. Your feet should be about shoulder-width stance with toes slightly pointing out. Curl your toes up. Puff your chest up when lifting up. Pull your shoulders back. Look forward during the whole lift. Keep your hands wider than your legs. Keep your arms straight. If you deadlift correctly, you'll feel most stress in your upper-back, glutes, and hams. Push from the heels. This automatically puts the weight on your heels. Squeeze your glutes. Bring your hips forward by pushing from the heels and squeezing your glutes hard. This prevents pulling with the lower back. The deadlift ends when your knees and hips are locked. No need to roll the shoulders or hyperextend the lower back.

Bringing the Weight Down. Don't lose time bringing the weight down. Do it controlled but not slow. The rule: hips unlock first, then knees. Chest up. Look forward. Neglecting to do both will make your back round. Keep your chest up, shoulders back, and look forward. Bar close to you. Keep the bar in contact with your thighs until it reaches knee level. It's friendlier on your back. First hips, then knees. Flex at the hips first to return the bar below knee level, then bend at the knees until the bar is on the floor.

USE LIGHT WEIGHT! TRY IT FIRST WITH JUST THE BAR WITH NO WEIGHT, THEN PUT A FIVE POUND WEIGHT PLATE ON EACH SIDE. AFTER YOU SUCCESSFULLY DO THE EXERCISE AT LEAST TWICE, YOU CAN MOVE TO TEN POUND WEIGHT PLATES ON EACH SIDE. You can also use dumbbells. Stand shoulders-width apart and have the weight in front of you. Check it out on the YouTube video below.

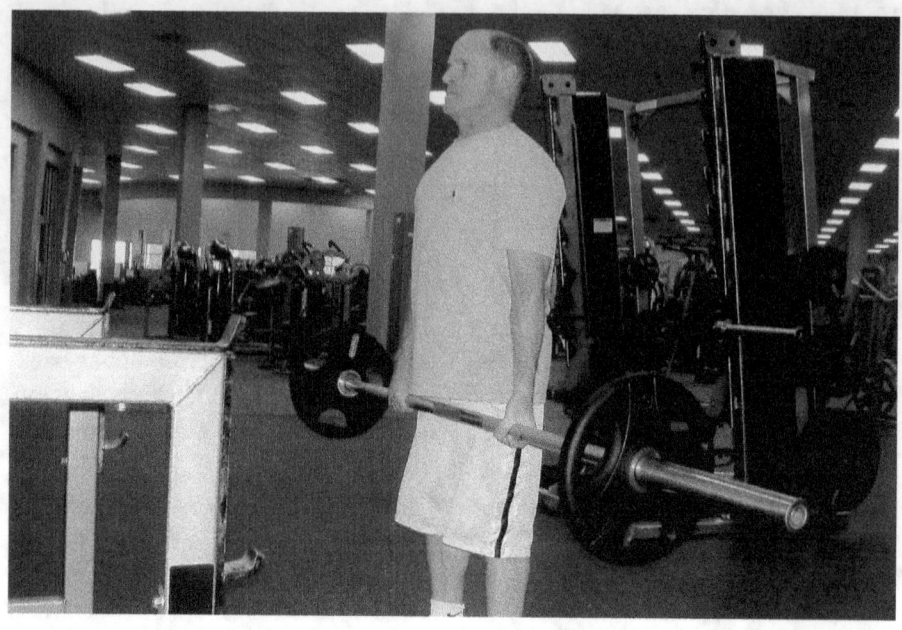

http://www.youtube.com/watch?v=cs-wOHN5tdw

(Do this exercise on a day you are not doing the superman exercise.)

Remember to do cardio for twenty minutes per day. Walking, cycling, stair master, elliptical machine, jogging, swimming, aerobics.

Tip 14 - Swim

Swimming is an excellent exercise on many levels. You get cardiovascular benefit, muscle strengthening benefit, and stretching. This is an excellent exercise to work all the muscles in the body. It can help you have a strong back. Gravity is not compressing the spine, the disc are not being compressed. The swimmer has to hold his/her body horizontal to the bottom; this works the core and back muscles. Swimming is a whole body exercise. It is not tough on the joints like aerobics or jogging.

Tip 15 - Yoga

Yoga is an excellent exercise system to keep your back healthy. Yoga has been practiced for thousands of years. Yoga helps with flexibility, strengthens muscles, helps with breathing, and is great for stress management. Yoga helps to strengthen postural muscles, the muscles that hold your body upright. Postural muscles become weaken from lack of use or injury. Yoga can help strengthen these muscles, helping the body to hold a proper posture. Once postural muscles are strong, activities like sitting, standing, lifting, and bending can be done more easily because the foundation of the body has been strengthened.

The breathing and meditation aspect of yoga helps to relax tight muscles and helps to release endorphins. Endorphins are chemicals your body releases that help you feel good and are natural painkillers. The breathing exercises help make sure the body is getting a lot of oxygen.

Let your doctor know you plan on taking yoga; there might be certain exercises that are not appropriate. If you have certain health conditions, make sure that the yoga instructor has worked with people that have had similar conditions. There are many types of yoga; make sure the class schedule is right for you and the class is not too difficult. Start out slow and let the instructor know you are a new student. I recommend that you take a few classes before signing up for a membership.

Tip 16 – Tai Chi

Yes Danielson, ancient martial arts can help you be healthier. Tai Chi is an exercise and ancient martial arts system that helps keep your back and your body healthy. Tai Chi has been done in China for thousands of years. Tai chi is a system of a series of slow movements that are performed in conjunction with specialized breathing. Tai chi helps with flexibility, balance, coordination, posture, strength, and stamina. Breathing helps to oxygenate the muscles and put the practitioner in a meditative state of mind.

Tip 17 – Pilates

Pilates focuses on the development and maintenance of core postural muscles. These muscles help keep the spine in alignment. Pilates is similar to yoga. Pilates has its roots in ballet and dance. And no, guys you don't have to wear a tutu. Unlike in yoga, special tables, bands, exercise balls, and equipment are used to do the exercises. Core muscles are the foundation for the other muscles in the body. People who do Pilates have excellent posture and rarely suffer from low back pain.

Tips While Playing Sports

Tip – 18 Ice is Nice

If you get hurt playing sports do this for the first twenty-four hours R.I.C.E. "R" stands for rest, rest the area. "I" stands for Ice. Ice the area for fifteen to twenty minutes, take the ice off for one hour then repeat up to three times. "C" stands for compression, compress the area. This means brace the area or wrap an ace bandage. "E" stands for elevation. Raise the area.

Tip – 19 Avoiding Tennis Injuries

Dr. Selinger's prescription for avoiding tennis injuries:

Inspect the court; make sure there are not leaves or water. You don't want to slip.

Wear the proper shoes, tennis shoes. Other types of shoes like running shoes can cause ankle and Achilles tendon injuries.

Warm up. This includes stretching hamstrings, quads, back, shoulders, neck, calves, and hips. Have a set routine that includes all the major muscle groups. Then warm up taking light strokes first. Then gradually increase the intensity of your swing.

Drink plenty of water; dehydration can lead to less blood flow to the muscles. If you dehydrate, you'll get tired and have cramps.

Get fit. To play any sport well, you need to be fit. Do some cardio exercise to build up stamina. Weight lifting can help to build the muscles you will use to play. If you are stronger, you'll be able to hit the ball harder and play longer.

Take lessons. Proper stroke mechanics will help prevent against many injuries.

Select the proper racket—make sure the grip isn't too small and that it's fitted to your skill level and your body. If the grip is too small, you'll probably over-use your wrist when you swing the racket, which will lead to wrist injuries.

You need time for the muscles to recover. Sleeping and rest is needed for muscles to heal; if you don't allow the muscles to recover, you will further injure yourself.

Tip - 20 Golf Safety

Low back injuries are the most common injuries for golfers. Golfers usually get injured from not warming up, overuse injuries, repetitive faulty swing mechanics, not being fit, or improperly fitted equipment (clubs and shoes).

Warm up and stretch the major muscle groups. Purchase a weighted driver, get a Momentus power driver. Gently swing the club back and forth; take a few easy short swings. Then gradually move into some longer swings. Begin your practice session with the sandwedge, then use the 9, 7, 5 irons and finish up with the wooden driver. Nice and easy swing.

Drink a lot of water while playing.

Stretch out, shoulder twirls, rotator cuff stretching, lat stretch, trunk twist, hamstring stretching. Check out this tip, on my blog on my website. I interview a golf pro that gives some tips on avoiding golf injuries.

Tip 21 - Avoid These Activities if you have a Herniated Disc

Jumping, running, bungee jumping

If you have a herniated disc, running or jumping can reproduce a compressive force on a weak disc, which can lead to further damaging the disc. The jarring motion reproduces trauma.

Bungee jumping can exert a sudden high velocity pulling affect on the spine; this type of force is not natural and can damage spinal structures. I recommend not doing this activity, but If you do this make sure you pack a diaper.

When skydiving, it's not the jumping out of the plane that injures your back, it's the landing. The landing exerts a lot of compressive force on the spine.

Tip 22 - Get a Chair with Good Lumbar Support

A chair with good lumbar support can help with low back alignment. Earlier, we talked about the natural inward curve that is located at the small of the back. A chair or pillow that puts light pressure on the curve in the low back helps muscles and ligaments sustain a proper sitting position longer and with less effort. A good lumbar chair or cushion helps preserve the natural low back curve of the spine. Even if someone has a strong low back, sitting in a seat for long periods of time with a poor lumbar support will likely affect that person's low back eventually.

Tip 23 - While Lifting Heavy Objects wear a Lumbar Support Belt.

Lumbar support belts or braces support the back while an individual is standing or walking. This helps give a hand to overworked or weak muscles. I highly recommend wearing a lumbar support belt if you have a low back injury, such as a herniated disc. Lumbar support belts are worn around the waist. It helps provide more stability for the low back when lifting objects. However, if it is worn all the time it can lead to a weakening of the low back muscles. I would recommend wearing the belt while doing a lot of lifting, after the work is done take the belt off.

Tip 24 - Jerry Seinfeld was Right.

"You have half a file cabinet under half of your ass." –Jerry Seinfeld.

I love the exploding wallet episode on Seinfeld, when George had a giant wallet and tries to justify why he needs to have a wallet that big. In the show, we find out George has back pain. Well, it's true an obese wallet can make you appear slanted and give you back pain.

An article published in January 2006 in the *New York Times* reported that sitting on a fat wallet could cause low back pain and sciatica (pain down the leg). The wallet puts pressure on the piriformis muscle—the sciatic nerve runs through this muscle. Compression of the muscles in the area of the wallet will cause those muscles to contract and compress the nerve. The person usually experiences pain down the leg, the buttock, or the hip areas. Also, sitting with the spine tilted on one side for prolonged periods of time can cause scoliosis, a lateral curvature of the spine. This induced scoliosis can lead to back pain and degeneration of the spine. Put the wallet in the front pocket or get a money clip.

CHAPTER 6

Ergonomics

Tip 25 - Working at your Workstation

It's a challenge to work on the computer without injuring your back or neck.

Your workstation should conform to you, not you conform to it. Your mom was right: slouching is not good. Slouching and other poor seating posture can lead to low back injury. A healthy body can only stay in one position for about twenty minutes. Change position after twenty minutes.

Standing on the job

First, you need to know what a good standing posture. Refer to the figure 3 on the right. If you are standing at work, this is the proper standing position:

- Align your head over the shoulders, head back
- Align the shoulders directly over the pelvis
- Tense the core abdominal muscles
- Tuck in the buttocks
- Bend knees slightly (so it's comfortable), place the feet slightly apart, with one foot positioned slightly in front of the other

Sitting at your workstation. Refer to the illustration below for proper seating position on the next page.

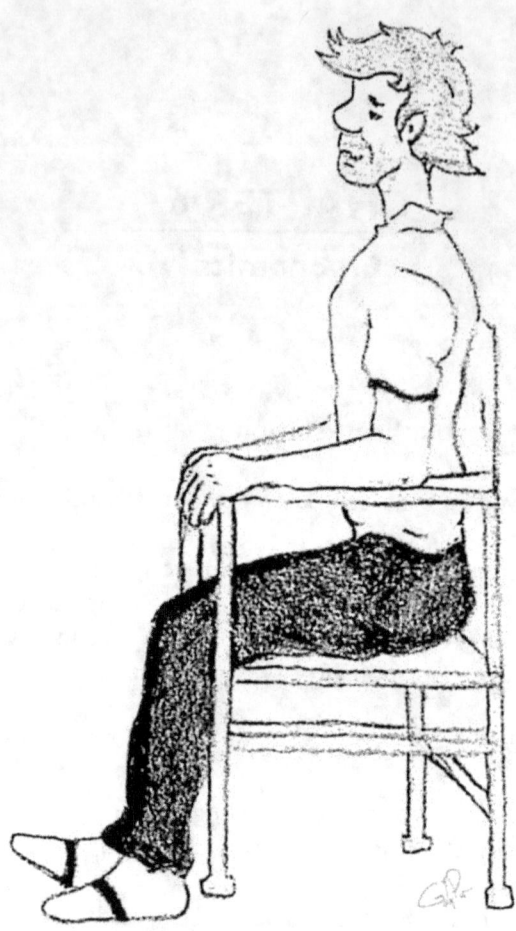

When sitting at the workstation, always take into account the height and weight of the worker when assessing proper seating at your workstation. Sit back in the chair, using the lumbar support. Don't hunch forward and sit on the front edge of the chair. Keep your head slightly back in alignment with your shoulders. Take periodic breaks and stretch hamstrings and low back. The work surface should be elbow high. Make sure the computer monitor is eye level. Choose the best height for the task you are doing and whether you are standing, or sitting on a chair or stool. Engineers, architects, artists and draftsmen may want a higher surface for drawing. Lower desk height is better for computer work.

The seat of the office chair should allow the work surface to be elbow high. Adjust the seat of the office chair so that the work surface is "elbow high."

Approximately a ninety-degree angle should be created at the knee when seated; if not, use a couple telephone books or a footrest to raise the knees level with the hips. The backrest of the office chair should push the low back forward slightly. If these adjustments cannot be adequately made with the existing office chair, a different make or type of chair may be considered.

Adjusting the height of the computer screen. Sit comfortably in the newly adjusted office chair. Close both eyes and relax. Then, slowly reopen them. The eyes should be able to look at the computer screen without having to tilt the head down or up. The screen can be raised using books or a stand if needed.

Tip 26 - Take a Break

Take a break from sitting. Sitting puts a lot of pressure on the lumbar disc. Sitting loads the lumbar disc three times more than standing. I recommend people take periodic breaks for a few minutes and stand, after sitting for an hour.

Tip 27 - Hauling Stuff

Proper material handling is key to avoiding back injuries.

We risk a back injury every time we handle objects, when we are lifting, climbing, pushing, carrying, pulling, or pivoting.

Lifting objects lower than your waist puts stress on the low back. Get as close to the load as possible, putting your feet diagonal if necessary, bend your knees, and keep your back straight. (Go to www.mylakeworthchiropractor. com for proper lifting video.)

When storing items, try to keep objects at waist level or higher, use lifts or shelves to help. The fewer times you have to bend to the floor, the better.

Carrying loads on your shoulder can make objects easier to carry. Sometimes carrying one load in each hand can balance the load and make carrying objects easier. For instance, you can carry one bag in one hand and an equally weighted bag in the other hand.

When climbing steps or a ladder use a "three point contact," meaning two feet and a hand must contact the ladder at all times. Don't be afraid of getting help from a coworker to help carry the load. And don't start texting people when you're on the ladder.

Pushing and pulling objects can also be hazardous to your back. Pushing is easier than pulling. I recommend pushing objects rather than pulling them.

While pushing or pulling objects, use both arms, shoulders, and bent legs to use the strength of your legs. Using handles, ropes, or straps can help. Properly used dollies and handcarts can save your back from injury. Or just pay someone else to do it. It will be cheaper than paying your deductible and co-pay.

Avoid bending, twisting, and lifting. These motions put a lot of stress on the disc in the back.

Tip 28 - Stand on Rubber Mats

Standing a lot on hard surfaces like concrete or tile can put a lot of stress on the low back. On hard surfaces there is little give, which means that the disc in your back will be absorbing most of your body weight. I recommend standing on a rubber mat to absorb the shock of the hard surface.

Tip 29 - Proper Sleeping Postures

A well-rested person is less likely to become injured than a person that is not getting enough rest. They are even less likely to complain...unless they live in Boca Raton. Muscles repair when we sleep; if you don't sleep, muscles can't repair. The best positions to sleep are in this order:

1) Back
2) Side
3) On your stomach, I don't recommend this one, unless you're
   sleeping next to Lorena Bobbitt

To relieve back pain while sleeping, try putting an extra pillow between your knees and then sleeping on your side or put the pillow under the knees and lay on your back. This can take some pressure off your back.

Tip 30 - Get a Firm Mattress

Personal preference is important. You need to be comfortable lying on the mattress, get a good night's sleep, and have proper support. I recommend medium to firm mattresses for my patients.

Waterbeds don't typically offer adequate support for your back. Plus, they are so seventies, just like handlebar mustaches.

The shoulders and hips should sink in a little bit; you don't want the mattress to be as hard as a rock.

Maintain the mattress by rotating the mattress 180 degrees every six months. I also recommend flipping the mattress over on the other side. If the mattress starts to sag or becomes indented in any area, you might need to get a new mattress, or a bra. (just kidding).

Tempur-pedic mattresses or memory foam mattresses can be great for some people. These are the mattresses you see the TV commercials, where there is a glass of wine on the mattress and someone is jumping on the other side of the mattress and the wine glass doesn't fall over. Not a great commercial I tried this and the wine glass did fall over, what a waste of wine. Memory foam molds to your body. I recommend calling local hotels and find out where they might have a memory foam mattress, try it for a night and see if you like it.

Tip 31 - Wear the Right Shoes

For every day walking around, I recommend wearing running shoes. Running shoes have high arches; high arches will support your foot better for straight walking. Many of my patients that have switched to wearing running shoes have less knee pain and back pain.

Now if you are going to play tennis or basketball, you're better off wearing a sneaker that has a lower arch support for side ways movement. If the arch is too high and you are walking sideways a lot, you will have a greater chance of spraining your ankle.

For a night out at the pubs, shoes with lower arches might be better in case you have a lot of sideways walking. You don't want to sprain your ankle.

Tip 32 - Avoid Wearing High Heel Shoes

They look good, even the ones that have see through heels, but they can be hazardous to your back. Women and men should avoid wearing high heel shoes. High heel shoes cause a lot of stress in the low back. If worn too much, high heels can lead to low back pain and to lumbar spinal misalignments.

Men wear high heels, too…they're called cowboy boots, and, yes, they can affect the low back the same way.

Tip 33 - Avoid Slippery Areas

People slip and hurt their backs all the time. Being aware of your surroundings can prevent an injury. Stop texting while you're walking around! Places where slip and falls occur frequently are supermarkets, fast food restaurants, parking lots, and other places that have good liability insurance. But seriously be careful, you can text later.

Tip 34 - Wear Orthotics

Orthotics are special arch supports you put in your shoes. Orthotics look like the inside sole of a shoe. They are contoured to support the foot to make sure you have a proper arch. Orthotics can help your feet and your posture. If your posture is maintained, it's less likely you'll have a low back condition. Some low back conditions can be caused from abnormal walking. Over time, even a slight abnormality can cause major problems. Orthotics can help with foot problems like fallen arches and a many other problems. When the foot is functioning properly, it can help the knees, hips, and low back function better. Custom orthotics might help to correct an abnormal walk and take stress and pressure off the back.

Tip 35 - Take Vitamins & Minerals

"The doctor of the future will no longer treat the human frame with drugs, but rather will cure and prevent disease with nutrition."

–Thomas Edison

The U.S. Department of Agriculture recommends that adults consume nine half-cup servings of fruits and vegetables each day for a reference 2,000-calorie daily diet. That's a lot. I recommend taking a multi-vitamin and fish oil supplements. Andrew Weil, M.D. said it best: "taking vitamins and supplements is like having insurance against the gaps in your diet." Taking supplements can help bridge the gap between what you get in your diet and what your body needs. Some people need more vitamins because they don't absorb the vitamins well. Women who are pregnant, older individuals, and people who have gastrointestinal disorders might require more vitamins.

It is important to make sure your body has the essential building blocks to build and maintain strong bones, muscles, and ligaments.

Vitamin D helps to build strong bones and teeth. Vitamin D is made in the skin with exposure to sunlight or by taking supplements. It is essential for the absorption to be able to absorb calcium. So people that are prone to osteo-porosis or don't get enough sunlight should take supplements to make sure they get enough Vitamin D. The daily allowance for people under fifty years old is 200 international units (IU), people over fifty is 400 (IU), and people seventy or over 600 (IU).

Vitamin C helps to increase calcium absorption for the bones. Helps to heal broken bones. Helps to decrease inflammation and helps with immune func-tion. Recommended dosage per day is 250 to 500 mg twice daily.

Vitamin B. Vitamin B1, B6, and B12 helps heal inflamed nerves and helps nour-ish nerves.

Vitamin E is an antioxidant that helps fight free radicals. When we have inflam-mation, a lot of free radicals are released. Vitamin E counters the free radical production. I recommend 400 IU daily.

Calcium and magnesium help promote bone growth. This helps to decrease osteoporosis. Calcium is a building block for bone growth. Magnesium helps to decrease muscle spasms. Calcium dosage is 600 mg daily. Magnesium dos-age is 250 mg daily.

Omega 3 is a fatty acid can help with immune function, cardiovascular func-tion, brain function, and help to reduce inflammation. There are so many reported beneficial effects of taking Omega 3 fatty acids.

Zinc helps decrease inflammation, and 30 mg twice daily is recommended.

Avoid soda because it has phosphorus, which can leach calcium from the bones and contribute to osteoporosis.

CHAPTER 7

Chores

Tip 59 - Snow Shoveling

The amount of snow you lift per cubic feet can vary to weighting from five to twenty pounds. Repetitively lifting that much weight, can cause injury. You should stretch out before you start to shovel the snow. When you shovel, keep your back straight and bend your knees when you lift. Space your hands apart. Try to shovel the snow and put it in front of you, and try to minimize twisting while holding the snow. Don't load the shovel with too much snow, take breaks, and pace yourself. Use a hard plastic shovel. Metal shovels are heavy, and you'll be lifting double the weight. When finding the right size shovel, it should be chest high. There are some new shovels that can minimize stress on your back, check out the "back savers" made by Lift with Ease. Dress properly and be careful of frostbite.

Check out this YouTube video:

http://www.youtube.com/watch?v=IVfWQfoaInc

Tip 60 - Mowing Lawn

Use a riding mower. Riding mowers push themselves; you don't need to push the mower. You will use less force to push the mower, and it's easier on your back and shoulders. Check out Honda's HRX2172VKA, John Deer JS36, and the Craftsman 37436. They are great riding mowers. Or just pay someone to cut the grass. I wish they had riding mowers that could write and finish books.

Tip 61 - Laundry

Use machines that are higher off the ground. Use the side loading machines that have pedestals. Pedestals raise the machines higher so you don't have to bend down as far. This can help save your back. Another recommendation I give patients who do have back conditions is, carry less laundry and make more trips to with smaller loads; don't carry as much. Another good back saving tip is use a hamper that has wheels.

Tip 62 – Vacuum

Keep your back straight and push the vacuum with your whole body. Move forward, stepping a push and step at the same time, so you are not just using you arms use your legs, too.

CHAPTER 8

Avoiding Injuries while Traveling

The only thing more annoying than sitting on a plane next to someone who can't stop talking is getting injured while traveling. Well sitting on the plane next to the bathroom isn't a picnic either. If you get injured while traveling, it can ruin your trip. Traveling can be hazardous to our backs. Many patients come into our office because of injuries acquired during traveling.

Tip 36 - Car Safety: Get a Safe Vehicle.

Many people injure their backs in auto accidents. Car accidents reproduce forces on the body that causes injuries to intervertebral disc, ligaments, nerves, bones, and muscles. The impact of the vehicle causes the vehicle to suddenly stop. Unfortunately, the occupants are still moving at the prior speed of the vehicle. Newton's first law states that a body in motion stays in motion. When you are traveling in a car at fifty miles per hour, your body is moving at fifty miles per hour. When the vehicle crashes, your body hits the steering wheel at the approximate speed the car was traveling just prior to the impact. There are other forces involved: the speed, mass, and direction of the other vehicle must also be taken into account. Seat belts help restrain the occupants in the car from going through the windshield or hitting the steering wheel. The neck cannot be restrained by the seat belt, but air bags can help reduce the impact of the head on the steering wheel or windshield.

When a car accident occurs, seat belts hold the back close to the seat, but a shearing force in the spine can be created while the seat belt holds the spine in place. This can cause a herniated disc, ligament tearing, muscle tearing, or even a fractured vertebra.

Some vehicles are safer than others. Driving a vehicle that has high safety ratings can decrease the changes of injury and death. In 2009, the Insurance Institute for Highway Safety rated the following vehicles the safest:

Large cars:

- Acura RL
- Audi A6
- Buick LaCrosse 2010 models
- Cadillac CTS
- Ford Taurus 2009-10 models
- Hyundai Genesis 4-door models built after 11/08
- Lincoln MKS
- Mercury Sable
- Toyota Avalon
- Volvo S80

Midsize cars:

- **Acura TL**
- **Acura TSX**
- **Audi A3**
- **Audi A4**
- **BMW 3 series 4-door models**
- **Chrysler Sebring 2010 models with optional electronic stability control**
- **Dodge Avenger 2010 models with optional electronic stability control**
- **Ford Fusion 2009-10 models with electronic stability control (optional in 2009, standard in 2010)**
- **Honda Accord 4-door models**
- **Lincoln MKZ 2010 models**
- **Mercedes C class**
- **Mercury Milan 2009-10 models with electronic stability control (optional in 2009, standard in 2010)**
- **Saab 9-3**
- **Subaru Legacy 2009-10 models**
- **Subaru Outback 2010 models**
- **Volkswagen CC**
- **Volkswagen Jetta**
- **Volkswagen Passat**
- **Volvo C30**
- **Midsize convertibles**
- Saab 9-3
- Volkswagen Eos
- Volvo C70

Small cars:

- Ford Focus 2-door models with optional electronic stability control
- Honda Civic 4-door models (except Si) with optional electronic stability control
- Honda Insight 2010 models with optional electronic stability control
- Kia Soul 2010 models
- Mazda 3 2010 models with optional electronic stability control
- Mitsubishi Lancer with optional electronic stability control
- Nissan Versa 2010 models with optional electronic stability control
- Scion xB
- Subaru Impreza
- Toyota Corolla 2009-10 models with electronic stability control (optional in 2009, standard in 2010)
- Toyota Prius 2010 models
- Volkswagen Rabbit 4-door models

Minicar:

- Honda Fit with optional electronic stability control

Minivans:

- **Honda Odyssey**
- **Kia Sedona**

Large SUVs:

- Audi Q7
- Buick Enclave
- Chevrolet Traverse
- GMC Acadia
- Mercedes R class built after 9/08
- Saturn Outlook

Midsize SUVs:

- Acura MDX
- Acura RDX
- Audi Q5
- BMW X3

- BMW X5
- Cadillac SRX 2010 models
- Chevrolet Equinox 2010 models
- Dodge Journey 2010 models
- Ford Edge
- Ford Flex
- Ford Taurus X
- GMC Terrain 2010 models
- Honda Pilot
- Hyundai Santa Fe
- Hyundai Veracruz
- Infiniti EX35
- Lexus RX 2010 models
- Lincoln MKT 2010 models
- Lincoln MKX
- Mercedes M class 2009-10 models
- Nissan Murano
- Saturn VUE
- Subaru Tribeca
- Toyota FJ Cruiser
- Toyota Highlander
- Toyota Venza
- Volvo XC90

Small SUVs:

- Ford Escape
- Honda CR-V
- Honda Element
- Mazda Tribute
- Mercury Mariner
- Mitsubishi Outlander
- Nissan Rogue
- Subaru Forester
- Toyota RAV4
- Volkswagen Tiguan

Large pickups:

- Ford F-150
- Honda Ridgeline
- Toyota Tundra

Small pickup:

- Toyota Tacoma

Tip 37 - Driving Properly

We spend so much time driving that our driving posture is important. When seated, the knees should be level with the hips. From the side view, your ear should be inline with your shoulder. Your shoulder should be inline with your hips. Look at the proper seating posture early in the book. . Don't bring your head too far forward—not only do you look ridiculous, you'll soon have neck and mid back pain. Lean back the maximum angle of the seat back to recline should be no more than thirty-five degrees from the vertical.k a little. Don't lean too far back;

Sometimes I recommend people who have a low back condition to put a pillow or lumbar support between the seat and the low back.

Sit at a comfortable distance from the steering wheel. The National Highway Traffic Safety Administration recommends approximately ten inches of distance between the center of the air bag cover and your chest. This serves to reduce injury from air bag deployment.

Tip 38 - Lifting luggage

"One time I went into a hotel, I asked the bellhop to handle my bag - he felt up my wife."

–Rodney Dangerfield.

When lifting anything heavy, always get as close as possible, bend your knees, and lift with your legs. When lifting carry on bags to the overhead compartment, bend at the knees lift with your legs. Place the bag first on the arm rest or the chair of the plane then lift it in the second stage and place it in the overhead compartment. As mentioned before, don't bend and twist while lifting.

Tip 39 – Wheels are Great

Buy luggage with wheels. It's so much easier to wheel the luggage around the airport than carrying it.

Tip 40 - Ask for Assistance

Don't be afraid to ask for assistance getting the bag into the overhead compartment. Believe me, if you get hurt, you'll regret not having asked for help.

Tip 41 - Ship your Bags.

Ship your bags ahead to the place you are staying at. I wish I could ship all my baggage. Call the hotel you are staying at and see if they can accept the package before you check in. If it is a business trip, you can ship the bag to the office you are going to visit.

Tip 42 - Check Your Bag at the Curbside Check In.

First, park next to "curbside check in" and check your bags, then park your car after you check your bags. The other option would be to take a shuttle or car service to the airport and have them unload your bag for you at "curbside check in." When you arrive at your destination, you can get assistance and have someone help you to your car from baggage claim. If you have a back condition this is the way to travel.

Tip 43 - Use a Back Pack

Back packs distribute the weight on your belongs across your shoulders and mid back, I would recommend getting a back pack, just don't over stuff it. That leads us to our next tip.

Tip 44 - Pack Less Stuff.

It is much easier to travel if you pack light. Pack clothes that are easy to match with everything, so you'll have many different combinations you can wear. For instance, if you have three shirts and three pants, make sure you can wear any of the pants with each shirt.

Tip 45 - Get Rid of Old Clothes.

Bring some old clothes that you can wear then leave on the trip and not bring back home. It will save you a trip to goodwill.

Tip 46 - Ice is Nice on Trips, Too.

Ice is not just for cocktails. If you can bring a mini cooler with ice packs, it could help to decrease inflammation. Leave ice on the area for fifteen to twenty minutes.

Tip 47 - A Lumbar Support Pillow can be Your Best Friend.

Place a small pillow, like the ones they have in the overhead compartment, (no not over the guy's face that's snoring and drooling next to you), put the pillow between the seat and your low back. They even have blow up lumbar supports. Sit with your shoulders back. This should be comfortable; if not, use a smaller pillow, rolled up clothing item, or towel.

Tip 48 - Tens Units are Great,

Tens units help to decrease pain by providing electrical stimulation to an area. Thanks to the terrorists, tens units are almost impossible to get on the plane. You might need a letter from a health care provider to be able to bring this device on board. Contact the airline prior to your flight and check to see what you need to do. Make sure you know how to properly use the device. Improper usage can result in burns or shock.

Tip 49 - Get an Aisle Seat.

Having an aisle seat will allow you to be able to easily get up and stretch. It can also allow you to walk around.

Tip 50 - Avoid Sitting in the Last Aisle

I have had bad luck while flying, and ended up having to sit in the back aisle. In most planes, the back aisle seats either don't recline at all or they recline very little. These seats don't recline and can be uncomfortable. As a bonus, they are usually next to the bathroom. Pack an air freshener.

Tip 51 - Request the Emergency Exit

This is the best seat in coach. It has the most legroom, and they fully recline. Book earlier because they book up fast.

Tip 52 - Recline

Sit back and lean back. This takes pressure directly off the lower back. The body weight is disbursed across more areas of your back.

Tip 53 - Drink Water

Drinking water helps with altitude sickness, and keeping muscles hydrated prevents cramping.

Tip 54 - Wear Comfortable Shoes

Travel with shoes that are easy to get on and off; this makes it easier to get through security with less chance of straining your back. If you're driving, keep your shoes on.

Tip 55 - Get a Letter from a Doctor.

Getting a letter from a doctor can help you get the accommodations you need: aisle seat, getting on the plane first, having someone help you with your bags. You'll get special treatment, and you don't even have to be on a reality show.

Tip 56 - Get some Rest

Go to sleep if you're flying. Use a "C" shaped neck pillow and a lumbar pillow. Sometimes if you bring a night mask and headphones you can tune out even the noisiest kid. Hopefully no kids start kicking the back of your seat.

Tip 57 - Wear a Lumbar Support Belt.

I mentioned earlier the benefits of wearing lumbar support belts. Lumbar support belts can be worn while sitting. However, you need to loosen the support belt so it is not too constricting, the belt should be comfortable and fitted around the abdominal area. Wearing a lumbar support belt while seated can help you if you suffer with back pain. Prolonged sitting puts a lot of stress and pressure on the lower back. Wearing a good lumbar support belt can help prevent muscle spasm. The belt gives weak back muscles a hand.

Tip 58 - Kids Back Pack Safety

Over 11,200 ER visits last year were reported due to backpack injuries. This has developed into a problem. It seems that our kids' backpacks have gotten bigger and heavier over the years. When kids are walking around with their backpacks, they have enough gear to ship out to Iraq. When we were kids, we had it easy: a few books, a couple of pens, and your "Stretch Armstrong man." Today, kids over-pack.

Reduce the loads these kids are carrying. Carry only the essentials.

The ABC's of backpack safety:

A. Appropriate weight 10-15% of child's weight
B. Both straps should be worn by the child, distributing the weight evenly
C. Carry about half of the amount of books

Make sure that the backpack is not too large; more stuff gets put in until the backpack gets full. Make sure the straps are wide and padded, the back of the backpack is padded, and make sure the backpack does not hang too low below the waist. This implies your child's pants are on his/her waist, not hanging below his/her butt. And to think...back in the day, people thought parachute pants were ridiculous.

CHAPTER 9

Wrapping It Up

Being healthy is partly a choice and partly genetics. Some people have bodies that can tolerate an unhealthy lifestyle. Everyone is different and has a different immune response to toxins in the environment. Some people are healthy to spite the bad choices they make. For example the late George Burns smoked cigars all the time and never got Lung cancer, while other people smoke for a short period of time and they get lung cancer. It doesn't seem fair. This is because genetically their bodies can handle smoking. But toxins are toxins and everyone that smokes is affected, some people might be affected more adversely than others. Maybe George Burns would have lived till 110 instead of a 100. We can really never know what could have been. If you chose to live an unhealthy lifestyle you are playing "Russian Roulette" with your body. Maybe the unhealthy lifestyle will rob you or 20 years.

Our bodies are constantly trying to adapt to the environment. But our bodies can only take so much abuse. If we feed the body garbage, and live a stressful lifestyle are bodies will eventually break down, even if you do have great genetics. People generally take their health for granted until they don't have it.

There is little you can do about your genetics, but you can make a conscious effort to take care of your body. The body will break down first at its weakest point. If our bodies are strong then we will be as healthy as genetically possible.

Take responsibility for your health. Your health is your responsibility. You can't outsource this responsibility to your spouse or your doctor. Only you decide what you will eat, drink, or if you will exercise that day. Living a healthy lifestyle is a choice you need to make. Ultimately, you need to take care of yourself.

If you are healthy, you'll require less medical service. Our health care system is going through major changes. The future is uncertain; I believe there are going to be cuts that will affect everyone. Don't rely on the health care system and insurance being able to take care of your needs. In the future, Medicare and major insurers will cover less of your healthcare expenses. Healthcare costs can put a person into bankruptcy. John Pottow, a professor at the University of Michigan, conducted a study that demonstrated a sharp rise in the number of bankruptcy fillings among the elderly due to healthcare cost. This can devastate a retirement account. Those who need less healthcare services will be richer. Many treatments, medications, and services will not be fully covered; this means higher out-of-pocket costs for consumers.

Take Action

This book should help to inform and inspire you to choose health. Hopefully, you start taking responsibility for your health today. Make choices that will give you the best chance of enjoying life to the fullest. A Healthy spine is part of a healthy lifestyle. If you take care of yourself, you'll have a better chance of living a high quality of life into your golden years. Be healthy for your children, grandchildren, brothers, sisters, parents, friends, or for your hospital room-mate. It's up to you what kind of life you want.

Prepare your body for the future, take stock in it, feed it, and make it strong. Create fun, healthy habits. If you do, you'll have taken your best shot at health.

www.ingramcontent.com/pod-product-compliance
Lightning Source LLC
Chambersburg PA
CBHW062110280526
45788CB00003B/1419